i

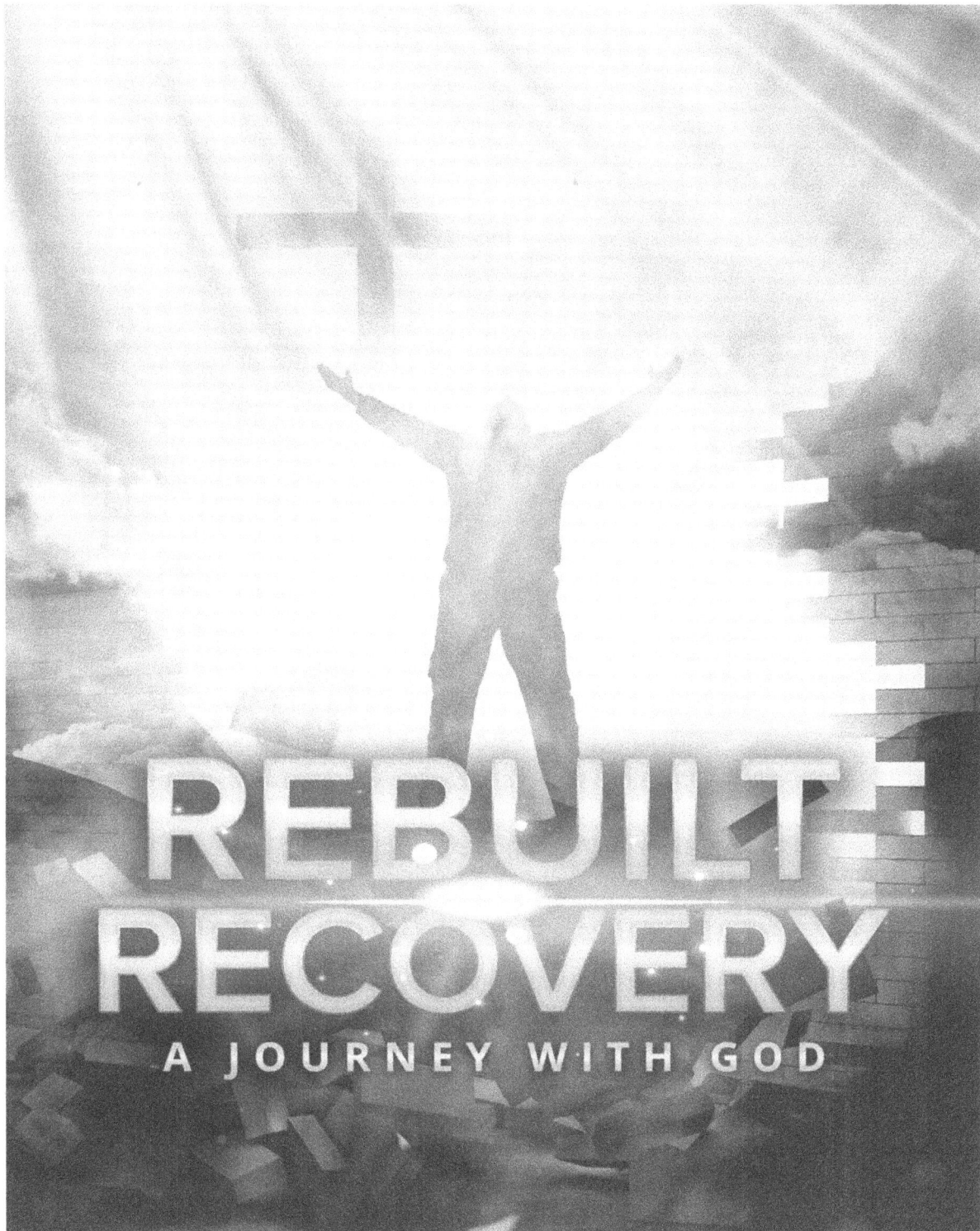

REBUILT RECOVERY

A JOURNEY WITH GOD

Glorious Hope Publishing

New Carlisle, Ohio

# Rebuilt Recovery

## A Journey with God

## Book 1— Getting Started

By: Heather L. Phipps

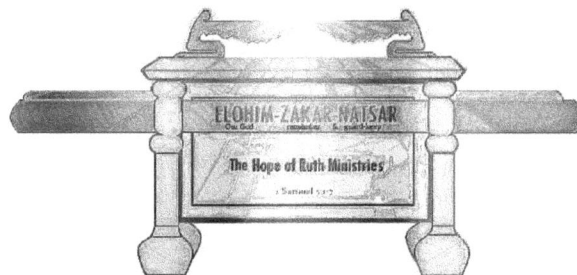

Rebuilt Recovery Is a Ministry of The Hope of Ruth Ministries Church

Glorious Hope Publishing

ISBN: 979-8-9852542-4-2 (Paperback)
Library of Congress Control Number: 2021922804

Glorious Hope Publishing
Hope of Ruth Ministries
307 Prentice Dr. New Carlisle, Ohio 45344
info@hopeofruthministries.com
www.hopeofruthministries.com

*Thank you to the following people
who gave their ideas, hearts,
and lives into making this book possible.*

Cindy Varghese

Summer Curtis

Alysha Allen

Justin Curtis

Annaka Schleinitz-Brooks

Jaycie Curtis

Camie Hawkins

Terri Allison

# Contents

# The Complete Rebuilt Series

# Rebuilt Recovery

### What Is *Rebuilt Recovery*?

*Rebuilt Recovery* is a tool to help people find recovery from their mental and emotional pain and suffering by dealing with the root causes of their issues.

Too often, attempts to heal mental health conditions address the symptom of the suffering without looking at the underlying cause. This is especially true with addiction. People often develop addictions in an attempt to mask pain from abuse, neglect, rejection, depression, grief, anxiety, etc. Treating the addiction without first treating the underlying causes feeding the addiction is only a temporary fix. When the person relapses, the problem intensifies, feeding guilt, shame, and feelings of failure that make the original problem even worse.

This is true of other mental disorders as well. OCD, depression, anxiety, schizophrenia, PTSD, or codependency are not the problem. They are the symptom of underlying issues. To treat the mental disorder without treating the cause will end in failure, and an eventual reoccurrence of the symptoms of the disorder.

**Rebuilt Recovery** is a tool that works in a cooperative effort with the Lord to permanently remove the underlying issues so people may have full healing and receive the joy and freedom promised in Scripture.

### What Causes Mental Illness?

Mental illness is complex. The truth is that there is no known, proven cause of mental illness. There is evidence to suggest that your genetic makeup may predispose you to certain mental ailments. This does not mean that you will develop a mental disorder, however; it simply means that it is more likely for you than for someone with a different genetic makeup.

It was once widely thought that the cause of mental disorders was chemical imbalances in the brain. It's true that the chemical balance of the brain does change with depression, anxiety, etc., but this theory, called the chemical imbalance hypothesis, is now widely dismissed by medical professionals. The chemical imbalances in the brain may cause the *symptoms* of these disorders, and medication can aid in easing the symptoms. The cause of the disorder, however, runs much deeper.

### What Causes Chemical Imbalances in the Brain?

Chemical imbalances occur when the brain produces natural chemicals called neurotransmitters. The job of the neurotransmitter is to help nerve cells communicate with one another. The way you think creates and reshapes the pathways of this intricate neuro-circuitry in your brain—in other words, your brain physically changes depending on how you are thinking. Your thoughts can literally change the physical structure of your brain. Mental illness is not genetic, but your genetic makeup may put you at a greater risk of developing a mental illness. The way you think about your experiences can activate your genes, so if you are predisposed to mental illness, your thoughts can activate those genetic factors.[1]

---

[1] More information on the science of thinking differently:

https://www.healthline.com/health/chemical-imbalance-in-the-brain

https://www.thebestbrainpossible.com/how-your-thoughts-change-your-brain-cells-and-genes/

https://www.psychologytoday.com/us/blog/bottoms/201611/what-is-cbt

https://www.psychologytoday.com/us/blog/what-mentally-strong-people-dont-do/201710/how-train-your-brain-think-differently

## How Do You Heal Mental Disorders?

### Physically

Medical professionals may prescribe medicine that works to compensate for the chemical imbalances in your brain as a temporary fix. They may also recommend vitamins, eating well, or exercise, which will improve mood and lead to a better quality of life.

Medicine is a Band-Aid® or a mask; it does not heal you. As your body adapts to medications, the dose must increase to create the same emotional state. Medicines must be used in conjunction with other treatment to be successful.

### Mentally

Counselors and therapists use a wide range of therapy techniques such as CBT (Cognitive Behavior Therapy) or CPT (Cognitive Processing Therapy) to change your perspective by training you to consider and reinforce positive beliefs and remove negative beliefs. When successful, there are proven long-lasting results. The solution is to restore the right way of thinking.

Therapies that change the way you think depend on reinforcing your beliefs. The positive thoughts become easier to believe as evidence reinforces the belief. If a belief fails the person, or he lacks evidence for it, destructive thoughts may again lead the person back into emotional instability. A person must base belief on unchangeable truth to effect a permanent change. The Lord is unchanging, and His truth will effect permanent change.

Many methods of treating mental illness often miss the spiritual component. We are not only physical and mental beings; we are also spiritual beings. We have the answer when we know Jesus and the Word.

### Spiritually

Churches attempt to address this problem through the concept of faith and works. If you believe enough—have faith—God will heal you. They instruct you in positive behaviors: quit sinning, serve more, live like Jesus, take authority, rebuke the enemy, put on the armor of God. However, churches often neglect the underlying physical and mental components of mental illness, relying only on the spiritual.

Christians have the answer, but many times they fall short in implementation. They often create an expectation of how God will move. People's faith tends to waiver when God does not meet their expectations. They may believe they are not good or spiritual enough for God to heal. Churches only fail if they address one part of the problem without the complete counsel of the Lord. **God's way of healing is found in Scripture and completely addresses mental, physical, and spiritual healing.**

Some Christ-centered recovery groups attempt to combine faith in God's word, living a Christian life, and spiritual warfare with therapy styles to change thought processes. They use Scripture to do this and achieve an excellent success rate. Yet these programs alone do not provide the complete foundational understanding of Scripture and God required to overcome addiction. This may lead people to a faith reliant on the program and not God. Full healing requires recovery and relationship.

### Complete Healing

Only with the Lord can you find complete healing. Complete and permanent healing comes when you:
- Discover the root of the problematic thinking
- Replace the negative thinking (the report of the enemy) with truth (the report of the Lord) based on God's unshakable and unchanging truth
- Reinforce the truth with evidence and translate the evidence into belief

*Rebuilt Recovery* Fills Gaps to Recovery through Scripture!

Complete healing does not mean that you will never experience difficult emotions or temptations. It means you will no longer suffer debilitating emotions or relapse because you have the tools and know-how to work through those difficulties, and you have the joy of the Lord in all circumstances!

## Why Is *Rebuilt* Different from Other Recovery Programs?

Christ-centered programs that focus on incorporating a spiritual and mental healing process are successful with those who are solid in their faith. However, these programs tend to neglect to instill a deep, foundational understanding of Scripture, leaving many still searching for the freedom and joy they were promised.

*Rebuilt* takes recovery to a whole new level. It is personal discipleship mixed with recovery. To be grounded in truth, you must know truth. *Rebuilt Recovery* is a process based on relationship. Why? Because relationship is the basis of everything God is and does. God is relational.

- God is Love (see 1 John 4:8). Love by its very definition requires an object. We are the object of God's love. He created us for the purpose of giving His love to us. Likewise, He desires that we give Him our love.

- God describes our relationship with Himself and other believers using relational language. He is our father, our husband. We are brothers and sisters in Christ, His bride, His child.

- God established people in families to teach us truths about Himself.

### The two greatest commandments fulfill all God's laws.

*Love the Lord your <u>God</u> with all your heart and with all your soul and with all your strength and with all your mind' and 'Love <u>your neighbor</u> as <u>yourself</u>. (Luke 10:27)*

- We are to first love God with our everything.

- We are to love others.

- We are to love ourselves. (This love is not self-centered, but is based on our identity in Christ.)

This is not love as defined by the world. This love It is sacrificial and defined by respect and admiration. This love is the foundational truth on which all Scripture builds. As we build a relationship with God, He teaches us this love, grounding our way of thinking in solid, unshakable truth, which comes from relationship with God. It is that relationship, which transforms our lives, not what we do or believe.

**Relationship with God changes our level of faith in Him** and provides us evidence of God. It gives us unshakable faith in His ability to provide, protect, guide, heal, and restore. We learn to trust through this relationship. Our faith activates God's power to move in our lives and remove our hurts, provide stability in chaos, and show us hope for the future God prepared for us.

**Relationships with others sharpen us, like iron sharpening iron.** Healthy relationships provide opportunities to forgive and make amends. God's Word shows us how to choose our relationships wisely, and how to love even people who seem unlovable. God made us for relationship. Nearly all trauma is caused by people, insecurity, or fear of a person's response: rejection, insults, abuse, negligence, crime, loss of people we love, etc. Learning how to relate to people gives us a fresh perspective on what people have done and helps us think about past events differently. Learning to relate to others helps us forgive them and truly release them from their wrong, thus giving us freedom.

**Relationship with self allows us to know ourselves as we truly are**. We must know ourselves. We must know where we flourish and fail, and we must examine the condition of our hearts. Even more than this, we must love ourselves. This sounds taboo, but Scripture does not say to love other people more than ourselves. God expects humility, but loving others as ourselves implies that we **must** also love ourselves. Because of our sin nature, we do not know how to love ourselves without it becoming a self-seeking kind of love. Scripture shows us how to do this. Loving yourself is seeing yourself through God's eyes, instead of through the lens of your experiences, failures, or your perception of another's opinion of you. It is loving the person God is creating in you as He transforms your heart. Loving yourself overcomes the not _____ enough feelings that come from shame.

## What *Rebuilt Recovery* is not

- *Rebuilt Recovery* is not a quick fix. It is a journey with God in a process of healing.

- It is not a 12-step program. It is not a program at all, but a tool.

- It is not responsible for your recovery. God does the healing through your journey.

- It does not take the place of doctors, psychiatrists, or therapists.

- It is not an alternative to medication and does not encourage you to stop medicines or go against any advice a medical care professional has put in place to stabilize you.

- Coaches are not licensed professionals, nor are they responsible for your choices.

- *Rebuilt* is not for people who are not serious about their journey or fully committed to do what God requires for success.

## What *Rebuilt Recovery* is

- A tool to guide you on a journey with the Lord through a process of recovery.

- A tool which transforms your lifestyle, drawing you nearer to the Lord and helping you build better relationships so you can relate to God, to others, and to yourself.

- A place of healing and trust, teaching you to develop trust and forgiveness.

- A tool that incorporates biblical principles of recovery, not just behavior modification, using the model of relationship and the "put offs" and "put ons" of Scripture.

*Where there is no guidance, a people falls, but in an abundance of counselors there is safety.*
*(Proverbs 11:14)*

## The Process

The crucial difference between this journey and other programs is that we approach healing through understanding relationships. The process is relational. This is your path to freedom:

### Relationship with God

- Learn that faith is more than simple belief.
- Deal with your doubt and denial.
- Learn to surrender and what that truly means.
- Learn realistic and biblical expectations of God and put to rest false expectations.

### Relationships with others

- Understand healthy relationships and their purpose.
- Understand the real meaning of love.
- Learn to have healthy friendships and families.
- Quit avoiding conflict and face your problems, biblically.
- Forgive others for the wrongs they have done against you, so you never have to struggle with them again.
- Learn that forgiveness is something you do once per transgression.
- Make amends for the wrongs you have done to others and experience freedom from your guilt.

### Relationship with yourself

- Examine the condition of your heart and learn three biblical "heart checks."
- Learn who you are, where your value and purpose lie, and the character of your God.
- Identify the original source of your emotions and your coping mechanisms.
- Learn to identify and distinguish the truth from the lies you are believing.
- Identify and remove the enemy's strongholds in your life, making the Lord your stronghold.
- Learn the things you must put off before putting on the Armor of God.
- Learn how to love the person God has created you to become.
- Confess the hurts and wrongs in your past and watch them lose their power over you.

### The Result

You will know your purpose and have hope for the future again. Your heart will be free from the burdens you have been carrying. You will experience new confidence in yourself and your God. Your faith will become unshakable. Your relationships (as much as it depends on you) will heal. You will handle other people's flaws and their rejection. You will know which people are good for your life and which are not. You will have compassion and love for others, greater than you have ever been able to experience before. You will have an entirely transformed life.

# Introduction

## Preparing For Your Journey

Welcome to a new season in your life! **This introduction lesson will teach you all you need to begin your journey.** The following lessons are divided into weekly increments to keep you moving and not overwhelmed. Do not be discouraged if you take longer or get stuck. You may require deeper thought or a better frame of mind to move ahead. Some weeks you may be motivated to complete more than one lesson. Go for it! This journey is yours. God and you set the pace, **but it is important to continue despite tough days**.

*Rebuilt* **is a tool** designed to guide you on a journey of healing with the Lord. Of course, there is no tool, guide, journey, program, recovery, ministry, counselor, preacher, or drug that can fix you. They may help you cope, but only the Lord can fix your brokenness.

**Your coach along this journey is** your support person, to encourage and strengthen you. You are not walking alone, but your coach cannot make choices for you or heal you. Restoration and healing require a relationship with Jesus Christ and the work of the Holy Spirit.

## Listen to the Right Report!

**The report of the enemy** will try to convince you not to attempt this journey with lies that feed your strongholds of fear, insecurity, and pride. "This will be the same as everything else." "This won't work." "I don't really need this." "I can't trust God to heal me." "I am okay as I am." There is another report, however. **The report of the Lord is truth.** The Lord tells us that He will not forsake us, He will break our chains, freedom is in Him, and by our faith we are healed.

| God's responsibility | Your responsibility | The coach's responsibility |
|---|---|---|
| ✓ Show you truth about Himself | ✓ Have faith, believe the Lord will work | ✓ Guide you through the questions |
| ✓ Show you the truth about yourself and your life | ✓ Be utterly honest with yourself, God, and your coach | ✓ Share Scripture, personal experiences and insights from their journey with the Lord, etc. |
| ✓ Love you where you are | ✓ See it through with complete commitment | |
| ✓ Heal your heart | | |
| ✓ Forgive your sins | ✓ Choose something different | ✓ Help you see yourself more clearly |
| ✓ Take your life's burdens and place them on His shoulders | ✓ Prepare to change your thoughts about the past, people, & life | |
| ✓ Remove your fear | | |
| ✓ Give you genuine joy | ✓ Be willing to submit everything to the Lord, and make changes | |
| ✓ Empower you | | |
| ✓ Strengthen you | | |
| ✓ Give you a purpose | | |
| ✓ Change your heart | | |
| ✓ Make you a new creation | | |

## What Happens When You Ask the Lord to Join You on Your Journey?

Have you ever heard the story of the prodigal son? It is a type-shadow that shows what happens when one of God's children returns to Him for help. The son did what he wanted, squandering his life and inheritance. He became so desperate that he returned to his father prepared to work as his servant. The father saw him coming and rejoiced, preparing his best to celebrate his son's return. **He accepted the son exactly as he was with open arms of love.**

Starting this journey tells God that you are coming home for help. Oh, how he rejoices! As soon as you begin, He jumps right in with you, walking every step of the way by your side. Regardless of your current relationship with the Lord, He will respond the same way.

Why is this journey necessary? Why does God not just heal everything? God is a gentleman. He will not force your hand or force His way into your life. He allows us to choose Him **and His help**. When we finally humble ourselves enough to ask, He and all the angels in heaven rejoice!

**Am I honestly ready to make a commitment to this journey, regardless of what it takes? \_\_\_\_**

**What may prevent me from making this commitment?**

_____

_____

**Am I prepared to trust God to do what needs to be done? \_\_\_\_\_**

**What makes trusting God difficult for me? _____**

*You can begin **even if** you hold on to some doubt. Your honesty, openness and commitment allow your coach to offer suggestions and encouragement.*

## Using This Book and Journal

You need a journal. You may use a decorative journal or a simple notebook designated for your *Rebuilt* journey. Some people journal on their computer, although we recommend printing journal pages to keep offline in case something happens to the digital files. Your journal entries will become an invaluable resource. You do NOT want to lose them!

Each lesson has questions for you to answer. Answer the questions as you read. You will discuss the answers when you meet with your coach each week. Use your journal or a separate notebook to record your answers. Write the lesson number and question number before the answer to make it easier to keep your place (i.e., 1.1).

**How to Use Your Journal**

- Write every day.
- Write your unfiltered thoughts to help sort through clutter in your mind.
- Write about meaningful events during your journey.
- Write about how the Lord is speaking into your life, and His blessings.
- Record your victories! They are vital to remember in hard times.
- Take notes on things to discuss with your coach.
- Write about additional tasks your coach gives along the way.

*Your journal is your second most important tool, after the Rebuilt books!*

## Boxes and Symbols

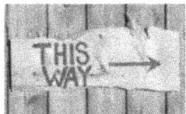

| | These boxes have thoughts or questions involving your coach. |

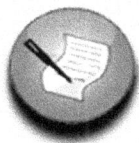

| | These boxes contain additional tasks for your journey. Do not skip these tasks! |

| | These boxes contain tips with additional information to help understand or implement the topic being discussed. |

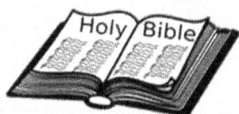

| | This icon indicates scripture important to understanding the current topic. |

| | These boxes have important points for you to consider. |

| | "These boxes contain interesting quotes" |

# Disclaimer

The information contained in the *Rebuilt for Life* (online course), *Rebuilt Recovery*, or *Rebuilt Website* is for general information purposes only. The content is not intended to be a substitute for professional advice, diagnosis, or treatment, rather it is intended as a supplement to it. Always seek the advice of your mental health professional or other qualified health provider with any questions you may have regarding your condition. It is your responsibility to inform your mental health professional that you are using a *Rebuilt* service to aid your recovery. Never disregard professional advice or delay in seeking it because of something you have read or heard in *Rebuilt* materials, website, or courses.

**Rebuilt coaches are not qualified counselors and do not take the place of certified professionals.**

The information is provided by *The Hope of Ruth Ministries* and whilst we endeavor to keep the information up-to-date and correct, we make no representations or warranties of any kind, express or implied, about the completeness, accuracy, reliability, suitability, or availability with respect to the website, books, online course, the information, products, services, or related graphics contained on the internet or print materials for any purpose. Any reliance you place on such information is therefore strictly at your own risk.

In no event will we be liable for any loss or damage including without limitation, indirect or consequential injury, loss, or damage, or any injury, loss, or damage whatsoever arising from loss of life, relations, property, data, or profits arising out of, or in connection with, the use of the *Rebuilt* website, *Rebuilt for Life*, *Rebuilt Recovery*, or *Rebuilt Coaches*.

Every effort is made to keep the websites up and running smoothly. However, *The Hope of Ruth Ministries* nor *Rebuilt Recovery* takes no responsibility for, and will not be liable for, the coaches, website, software, or course being temporarily unavailable due to technical issues beyond our control.

## COPYRIGHT NOTICE FOR SUPPLEMENTAL MATERIAL

## EXTERNAL LINKS

Through the *Rebuilt* websites and courses, you may link to other websites, which are not under the control of *Rebuilt* or *The Hope of Ruth Ministries*. We have no control over the nature, content, and availability of such sites. The inclusion of any links does not necessarily imply a recommendation or endorse the views expressed within them.

# Serenity Prayer

God, grant me the serenity
to accept the things I cannot change,
the courage to change the things I can,
and the wisdom to know the difference.

Living one day at a time,
enjoying one moment at a time;
accepting hardship as a pathway
to peace;

taking, as Jesus did,
this sinful world as it is,
not as I would have it;
trusting that You will make
all things right
if I surrender to Your will;

so that I may be reasonably happy
in this life
and supremely happy with You
forever in the next.

Amen.

Reinhold Niebuhr

## Support and Help

You are beginning a new journey with the Lord—most likely, a journey unlike any you have taken before. The Lord can help you all on His own, but that is not His design. God created us to need one another. In His infinite wisdom, God knows when we support others, not only can we guide them, but it also helps us to grow.

*As iron sharpens iron, so one man sharpens another.*
*(Proverbs 27:17)*

Your coach will guide you and commit to be there when the road gets bumpy, but additional support is a significant benefit. Accountability partners will keep you on the ideal track and can be available when your coach is not.

## The Right People Make All the Difference!

**It is important to bring the *right* people along for your journey.** Those who accompany you must have your best interests at heart, and trust is essential. The wrong person can lead you astray or encourage you to quit when things get hard. Someone who is judgmental may tear you down and prevent you from being entirely honest with yourself and your coach. Codependents may develop animosity toward your walk as the chains of codependency break.[2]

### Family and Friends

Long-standing relationships often have a familiarity that quenches objectivity. It is not always a good option to take close friends or relatives with you on this journey. The people in Jesus' hometown rejected him. To them, he was a mere carpenter's son. They could not accept that Jesus was more than they perceived Him to be.

*And Jesus said to them, "A prophet is not without honor, except in his hometown*
*and among his relatives and in his own household."*
*(Mark 6:4)*

While you are not claiming to be a prophet, you *are* beginning a transformational process in your life. Not everyone will be open to seeing the changes in you.

### Choose an Accountability Partner

An accountability partner is an important part of your journey. This is a trusted person who you respect and will be honest with. They must be able and willing to hold you responsible for your journey and keeping on track with your recovery. You must be willing to listen to their counsel, therefore they must be someone who will offer wise, helpful advice and not lead you to temptation. They must be willing to be contacted when you are struggling, even at inconvenient times. It is important to use care when choosing an accountability partner.

---

[2] Codependency is when a person in a relationship controls and manipulates another or depends on the other's needs or control.

Look for the following qualities in an accountability partner:

- Does this person encourage you and lift you up to believe you can be more?

- Does this person have a sincere desire to see you succeed?

- Do you trust this person enough to tell them your innermost secrets? Are they reliable to keep their word?

- Does this person listen well and try to understand you, or do they insist that you agree with their perspective?

- Does this person have a genuine and mature relationship with God?

- Does this person challenge you?

- Does this person have the fortitude and commitment to stand by you in difficult situations?

List some people who might make good accountability partners.

_____

_____

**Narrow your options**
If you can answer "yes" to any of the following questions about someone you are considering, they should *not* be your accountability partner.

- Does this person gossip or talk about others? If so, they will talk about you also, given the right circumstance.

- Will this person simply agree with you instead of speaking truth you will not want to hear?

- Does the person assume your motives or make comments such as "You always do_____" or "You never_____"? Do they judge your actions because they "know how you are"?

- Will a change in you affect your relationship in a negative or unhealthy way?

- Does this person demean or place guilt on you?

- Does this person create doubt in you and sabotage your success?

- Is this person jealous or threatened by your achievements?

- Is this person argumentative, unable to be wrong, or do they assume they know better than you do?

Write your choice for an accountability partner below.

_____

## Ask Someone to Be Your Accountability Partner

Contact the people you chose as potential accountability partners and ask them to come alongside you on your journey. Discuss the following points so they clearly understand what you expect from them.

- You are asking for a commitment to keep you on track and offer support through a challenging year-long journey.

- Sometimes you will need no accountability. Other times you may depend on them daily.

- Your needs may change throughout your journey.

- If you are struggling, you may need them at an inopportune time.

**Do not be discouraged if the person you approach refuses, or if you do not know anyone who would make a good accountability partner.** If the person you chose does not agree, that is okay. The Lord can bring someone along who is a good fit.

## You Are in Charge of Your Journey and Who Gets to Be Part of It!

Sometimes a coach or accountability partner relationship does not work out. This is nothing to worry about. While it is not recommended to leave your coach, if you have trouble relating well with him or her you may ask for someone else. If you are not comfortable with the people supporting you, it will be difficult to succeed.

- Your accountability partner or coach should understand it is not personal if you choose another to walk with you; it is where you are on your journey.

- Do not fear hard feelings when changing a member of your support team.

- Many things can change in a year! Personal situations may prevent someone from being a quality coach or accountability partner. It is better for them to step aside if they cannot be available and consistent.

- You are not required to explain your reasons for requesting a new coach or accountability partner.

- If you fire your coach or if your coach steps away, he or she will help find another to complete your journey with you.

** Coaches are not obligated to fulfill a commitment to people who do not put forth effort, are argumentative, or resist change. These attitudes make a journey ineffective and steal time the coach could spend helping someone ready for the journey. In this situation, a coach will recommend continuing the journey at a later time.

# Your Support Team

*Copy this page or ask your coach for a copy. Let it remind you to reach out to your support team when you are struggling. Keep it on your refrigerator, desk, or somewhere you will often see it, and keep your coach's information in your phone, wallet, or purse.*

**If you do not have an accountability partner yet, leave this section blank until you find one.**

## My *Rebuilt* Coach

| | |
|---|---|
| **Name:** | |
| **Number:** | |
| **Email:** | |
| **Facebook or Other Means of Contact:** | |
| **Preferred Contact Method:** | |

## Accountability Partner

| | |
|---|---|
| **Name:** | |
| **Number:** | |
| **Email:** | |
| **Facebook or Other Means of Contact:** | |
| **Preferred Contact Method:** | |

## Accountability Partner

| | |
|---|---|
| **Name:** | |
| **Number:** | |
| **Email:** | |
| **Facebook or Other Means of Contact:** | |
| **Preferred Contact Method:** | |

# Manage Your Time

Before starting *Rebuilt*, consider how you manage time to prevent becoming overwhelmed by the commitment.

Every purchase has a positive or negative return and a dual cost: the amount spent on the purchase and the hidden cost of everything you cannot get with the money spent. You receive a **positive return** as the property value increases in your home. However, the moment you drive away in a new car, its value depreciates, giving you a **negative return**. A losing lottery ticket is a **total loss**, leaving nothing to show for the money spent. It robbed you of your investment.

> Life's currency is time and energy, and like monetary currency,
> there is a dual cost and return when spent.

Time and energy are your most precious resources. Time is finite and irreplaceable; if we waste it, we cannot regain it. Energy makes time productive. As time passes, less energy is available. When your energy depletes, your time becomes unproductive. You spend more time accomplishing less.

## Understanding Wise Investments of Time and Energy

Read the definitions below to familiarize yourself with the terminology:

- **A Return** refers to positive or negative impact from investing time or energy.
- **A Positive Return** is when our effort adds an element of quality, surplus of energy, or redeems the investment for our benefit.
- **A Negative Return** brings harm to us or others, leaving us worse off for our effort.
- **Robbed of Time/Energy** implies an investment that steals time or is a complete loss. This includes mind-numbing activities like social media or television, non-productive time spent daydreaming or worrying, and investing time in someone who does not reciprocate or benefit from your investment.

We spend time and energy in four areas. To learn more about these four areas, read the descriptions below and answer the questions.

1. **Physical Investment** — Our activities are an obvious investment of time and energy. Exercising, walking, cleaning, cooking, working, traveling, sleeping, eating, or being sick, all cost time and energy. Physical investments such as laughing, crying, and fits of rage may also have an emotional investment such as joy, grief, and anger. This is a dual investment. Many times, our physical investments **return a positive benefit**. We exercise and our bodies become stronger. We go to work and earn money. When we help another, we receive joy. Sometimes, our physical investments give us a **negative return**. We fall behind when we waste time doing the wrong things. We lose opportunities when we are not wise in how we spend our time. Negative actions, such as yielding to addiction or gluttony of food or pleasure, provide a negative return to our health, our mental and emotional state, and even our wallets.

### Questions to Ponder

1) Consider what you do. What are your greatest physical investments?

2) What is the time and energy cost of your physical investments?

3) Describe the negative returns on your physical investments.

4) What positive returns result from your physical investments?

5) In what ways do your physical investments rob you of time and energy?

2. **Emotional Investment** — Emotions influence our investment of time and energy into people, dreams, goals, grudges, and ourselves. We may spend a great deal of time and energy fighting, denying, or avoiding emotions. Emotional investments may bring joy and a sense of worth, or leave us drained with rage, grief, and sadness, as hidden violations and unforgiveness fester in our hearts.

### Questions to Ponder

6) What are your emotional investments?

7) How do your emotional investments spend time and energy?

8) In a typical week, how often are your feelings negative? How often are they positive?

9) Do your emotional time and energy investments have a positive or negative return?

10) How do your emotions steal your time and energy?

3. **Mental Investment** — Many things require a mental investment of our time and energy: thinking, worrying, planning, researching, studying, writing, daydreaming, reading books, watching videos, or playing games. Dwelling on negative or ignoble things can drain our energy and rob us of our time or give us a negative return on our time. However, meditating on things of the Lord—His blessings, purpose, and future—can give us the positive returns of hope, encouragement, and motivation. When we rest our mind in the Lord, He renews our strength and energy.

### Questions to Ponder

11) What are your mental investments?

12) How do your mental investments spend your time and energy?

13) Is your thinking mostly positive (hopeful), negative (pessimistic), or neutral?

14) What thoughts give you a positive or negative return?

15) What thoughts give you no return, robbing you of your time and energy?

4. **Spiritual Investment** — A spiritual life requires time and energy. We seek spiritual wellbeing to find meaning, purpose, and security in life. Investing time and energy in a relationship with God fills our spiritual needs. The Lord renews our energy, gives us rest, and redeems our time. When we seek to fill our spiritual needs from different sources—such as nature, self, money, or idols—our investment returns void or empty of meaning. Our drive to seek purpose and meaning exhausts our energy.

> ## Questions to Ponder
>
> 16) How much time and energy do you spend in prayer, devotion, church, witnessing to others, worship, Bible reading, or meditating and listening to the Lord?
>
> 17) What other spiritual influences are in your life? (E.g., horoscopes, fantasy, spiritualism apart from the Lord, books, movies, etc.)
>
> 18) What is the return on your spiritual investments? What percentage of your return is negative, positive, or both?
>
> 19) Are there any negative influences you allow to take up your spiritual time and energy? Are you aware of the impact and cost to you?
>
> 20) How do spiritual investments steal your time and energy?

Now, consider this next set of questions to help you break down the cost of your time and energy and how that cost affects your life.

> ## Questions to Ponder
>
> 21) Estimate the percentage of your time spent in each category. (For example: 40% Physical, 25% Emotional, 30% Mental, 5% Spiritual.)
>
> 22) Estimate the percentage of your energy spent in each category.
>
> 23) What investments give a positive return?
>
> 24) What are the benefits of the positive returns you identified?
>
> 25) What investments give a negative return?
>
> 26) What harm comes from the negative returns you identified?
>
> 27) Which investments leave you robbed, unable to identify a return or loss?
>
> 28) What losses have you identified resulting from the way you invest your time and energy?
>
> 29) How are you spending more time and energy than you have available to give?
>
> 30) How could you invest less time and energy in the things that rob you or give a negative return?
>
> 31) How could you invest more time and energy in the things with a positive return?
>
> 32) Is there any investment that causes a negative return or loss, which you can invest differently to create a positive return?

# Let's Begin

God is ready to embark on this journey with you. Give Him your trust one day at a time and watch as He increases your faith. When experiencing hard times, do not fear failing or that you lack the faith to succeed. Remember your commitment and move forward anyway. It is in these times that the Lord proves Himself faithful. This journey will cover steep hills and deep valleys, but you never walk alone. For every difficult moment, there is an equally exciting victory!

## Say a Prayer

Would you embark on a trip with friends without first discussing it? Of course not! This is no different. Take a moment to pray, asking the Lord to accompany you on your journey. In reality, you are not inviting Him to come with you, but requesting to go with Him. He is the one leading your journey.

Are you unsure how to pray? *Rebuilt* does not script prayers, as they must be a genuine reflection of your heart. If you struggle to find the words, consider the suggestions below to guide your prayer:

- Thank the Lord for your blessings and this opportunity.
- Repent and seek forgiveness if something weighs on your mind.
- Commit to seeking healing in His ways.
- Ask the Lord to reveal Himself through this journey.
- Ask the Lord to search your heart to uncover any denial.
- Share any doubt, lack of faith, or unbelief with the Lord.
- Pray regarding any concerns you have about beginning this journey.
- Ask the Lord keep you accountable, honest, and committed.

# Ready,
# Set,
# Begin!

# Introduction to Book One

## Prepare the Way

As with any journey, you must prepare before you leave: Plan the route, pack the right supplies, and choose your travel companions. It is the same way on a spiritual journey!

**Plan Your Path**
Your path is set before you. Consider this guide your GPS.

**Pack for the Journey**
You will travel light. All you need is a Bible, this guide, a journal (or two or three ...), and pens or pencils.

**Your Travel Companions**
You will travel with the Lord, whose spirit will minister to you and teach you throughout your journey, and with your coach, who will be there to keep you focused on the Lord and give some encouragement along the way. Once you get started, you may make a pit stop and ask one or two trusted friends to come along on the journey. They can give additional support and help keep you accountable.

**Plan Adventures and Sight-seeing**
There will be many destinations along the way, and it will be the greatest adventure of your life. You will see many sights as your eyes become opened to the truth. But as with everything, there are guidelines to follow:

- Be completely honest with yourself, your coach, and God. The road becomes bumpy and treacherous when you break this rule.
- Never give up. Quit the journey early, and you may end up stranded in the wilderness without a ride home.
- Do not isolate yourself. You can easily get lost in unfamiliar territory if you pull away from your coach or from God. You do not want to be stuck in the wilderness!

**Method of Transportation**
One step at a time. You can walk through the books at your own pace, just do not stop moving. Your coach will go over your answers to the questions in the book, your journal (if you want to share), and answer questions along the way.

- Meetings with your coach are confidential, so you can be free to share whatever is on your mind. (Your coach will discuss this in more detail with you).
- Pray before working through the books and listen for the Lord.
- Each day, journal about your feelings, concerns, or what the Lord is teaching you.

# Chapter One

## Faith

# Lesson 1 — Defining Faith

**Questions to Ponder**

**1.1)** To begin a journey with the Lord requires faith. Before we look at what the scriptures say, take a minute and write in your notebook or journal what you believe faith is, and what it requires of you.

**1.2)** Is a belief that Jesus existed, died, and rose again the only thing required for salvation? If your answer is no, then explain what else is required.

**1.3)** In your understanding, what does it mean to know Jesus?

## What Does Scripture Say?

Scripture uses the words *faith* and *belief* similarly, but when we consider belief, we often see it from a narrow perspective. Let us look at the most famous passage in all of Scripture, John 3:16:

> **For God so loved the world, that he gave his only Son, that whoever believes in him should not perish but have eternal life.**

This verse by itself seems to say that all salvation requires is to believe that Jesus existed, and that He died and rose from the grave. Some view anything else as works and not a requirement for salvation. However, no single verse of Scripture was ever intended to be the only word of God on a matter. We must consider the whole counsel of God. The Lord expresses that there is more to relationship with Him than the simple belief Jesus exists when he says this:

> **Many will say to Me on that day, "Lord, Lord, did we not prophesy in Your name, and in Your name cast out demons, and in Your name perform many miracles?" And then I will declare to them, "I never knew you; depart from me you who practice lawlessness." (Matthew 7:21 – 23)**

The Lord describes people who believed in Him, even used His name to perform miracles—yet Jesus says to them, "I do not know you." Realizing that the name of Jesus has power and knowing Scripture are not sufficient to save us. We must **know Him**.

## What Does It Mean to Believe? What Is Faith?

Hebrews 11 tells us what God means when He speaks of faith in Scripture. Faith is confidence or **trust** in what our senses cannot perceive. It is assurance of our hopes.

> **Now faith is confidence in what we hope for and assurance about what we do not see. (Hebrews 11:1)**

We all have had experiences where we realize God has come through for us, and times we feel He disappointed us. Many times, our disappointment comes because we cannot see the whole picture. We cannot understand why our prayers were not answered the way we assumed they should be answered. This can cause us to doubt God.

> Do not worry if you struggle to answer the lesson questions. Mistakes are where learning happens! Sometimes we cannot know the answers, or the answers come later. The important thing is to understand that just because we do not have all the answers, we **can** still have full confidence in our God.

## What Faith Looks Like

We know that **without faith it is impossible to please God** (Hebrews 11:6). The rest of Hebrews 11 shows examples of the attitudes and actions of faith. Unwavering trust allows us to be obedient to God even when, in our own wisdom, we cannot make sense of His commands.

### Read Hebrews 11

#### Questions to Ponder

1.4) When, if ever, did you put your trust or hope in God for a situation that you could not control or understand?

    a. Was the outcome what you thought you wanted? Was the outcome better or worse than you expected? How did this situation change your level of trust in God?

    b. Did the outcome of the situation disappoint your expectations? How did this change your level of trust in God?

1.5) Are you willing to look at situations in which God did not answer your prayers the way you wanted from a new perspective? Can you see any other possible reasons for the way the Lord responded to your prayers?

## Examples of Living a Life of Faith

The people mentioned in Hebrews 11 are examples of living a life of faith. They **lived by faith** until they died. Even if they **did not see the result** of the promise, they set their minds on eternity and were Kingdom-minded. **God was unashamed** of them and counted them as righteous because of their faith. Their faith was not a simple belief, but a faith that produced obedience.

Each person in Hebrews 11 had sin and major life mess-ups, yet God calls them all righteous.

- Noah became so drunk one night that his son Ham caught him passed out and naked.

- Abraham, the "father of our faith," falsely claimed that his wife was his sister to escape harm.

- Moses murdered an Egyptian, feared speaking to pharaoh, and had a temper problem.

**From Hebrews 11 we learn that faith is**

- A belief that Jesus exists

- An earnest seeking after Him

- Demonstrated through sincere offerings

6

- The fear of the Lord
- A knowing that God is a God of His word, trusted and respected
- Obedience, even when we do not understand the why
- To go where God sends us
- To believe God is faithful to us, that his word is true **for us**
- To know God's promises **will be fulfilled**, even if we do not see the result in our lifetime
- To stay hopeful because we set our minds on the things of the Kingdom, of eternity, not things of this world
- To suffer and persevere with Christ
- Not fearing the world's ridicule, imprisonment, even death, because our faith is in that which is eternal

## Faith is relational!

### Questions to Ponder
1.6) Do you ever think your sin may keep God from helping you? Is this truth?

1.7) Looking at the list from Hebrews 11, in which areas is your faith strong?

1.8) Are there areas where you cannot trust God?

## Faith Activates God's Power

**Our faith, as defined by the Word of God, moves the Lord to activate His power in our lives.** The Lord guarantees that when we trust and submit our journey to Him, He **will** change our lives and heal us from hurts and strongholds keeping us stuck. Sometimes it is hard to trust, and this allows doubt to creep in.

> *But let him ask in faith, with no doubting, for the one who doubts is like a wave of the sea that is driven and tossed by the wind. For that person must not suppose that he will receive anything from the Lord; he is a double-minded man, unstable in all his ways. (James 1:6 – 8)*

## Trust Is an Act of Love

Trust is a gift, which is an act of love. When we give God our trust, we are showing him love. It is an act of love because trust is sacrificial. To give even that small amount of faith makes us vulnerable, because the one to whom we are giving faith may fail us. We may get hurt. Faith is a selfless act of love and trust, and the greatest gift we can give God. We do nothing in our own power; the only thing we have control over is our choices. We cannot even choose God without Him drawing us in.

> *No one can come to me unless the Father who sent me draws him.*
> *And I will raise him up on the last day. (John 6:44)*

The choice we really need to make is whether we will trust the Lord. Even a small amount of trust will do a lot. When we learn about Christ and dig into His word, we make a choice to believe.

*So faith comes from hearing, and hearing through the word of Christ. (Romans 10:17)*

<u>Questions to Ponder</u>

1.9)  How do you struggle with doubt?

1.10)  What are your Bible study habits? Do you trust the Word of God?

1.11)  List any questions about God or the Bible that are a stumbling block to your faith.

1.12)  Are you willing to give the Lord an opportunity to prove He is trustworthy? What would that look like for you?

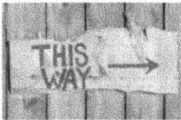

Work with your coach on your tough questions! Do not be afraid to ask your coach anything. If they do not know the answer, they will help you find it! Did you do the Time Management exercise in the Getting Started section? Review it with your coach!

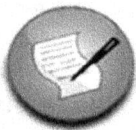

- Make it a habit to start each lesson in this workbook in prayer. Pray each morning about this journey you are taking.
- Ask to walk with the Lord throughout your day.
- Ask the Lord to guide you as you answer the questions in your notebook.
- Pray each evening about your day. Listen for the Lord to give you understanding. Write about it in your journal.

# Chapter Two

# Deal with
# Your Doubt

# Lesson 2 — Dealing with Doubt

No person increases our faith—not a pastor, mentor, or even ourselves. It is the Lord who gives the increase when we reach out with the smallest seed of faith.

*So neither he who plants nor he who waters is anything, but only God who gives the growth. ... You are God's field, God's building. (1 Corinthians 3:7,9)*

The apostles realized this and asked the Lord to increase their faith.

*The apostles said to the Lord, "Increase our faith!" And the Lord said, "If you had faith like a grain of mustard seed, you could say to this mulberry tree, 'Be uprooted and planted in the sea,' and it would obey you." (Luke 17:5 – 6)*

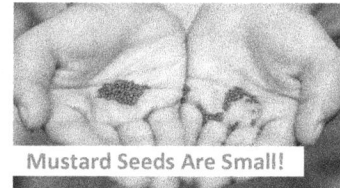

Mustard Seeds Are Small!

Jesus tells them that if they had even a little amount of faith (a mustard seed is very tiny), they could do the impossible. In other passages, Jesus scolds his disciples for not having enough faith. Yet in each case, He is telling them to simply believe. You can know something is true in your head, but believing it with all your heart is far more difficult.

We already know that faith comes by hearing the Word, so studying Scripture is a great place to start. **After all, how do you trust in a God you do not know?**

> ## How does faith grow?
> - By reading the Word
> - Through testing and trial
> - With prayer

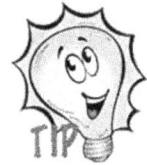

## Opportunity to Use Our Faith

God will give us opportunities to use our faith, testing our faith in trials. When everything is going well, it is easy to have faith in God, but the true demonstration of our faith is when the trials come. Do we trust God, put it in his hands, and believe for a victorious outcome, or do we try to control matters ourselves and thus fall into worry, panic, or fear?

*In this you rejoice, though now for a little while, if necessary, you have been grieved by various trials, so that the tested genuineness of your faith—more precious than gold that perishes though it is tested by fire—may be found to result in praise and glory and honor at the revelation of Jesus Christ. (1 Peter 1:6 – 7)*

*Count it all joy, my brothers, when you meet trials of various kinds, for you know that the testing of your faith produces steadfastness. And let steadfastness have its full effect, that you may be perfect and complete, lacking in nothing. (James 1:2 – 4)*

Of course, we can pray for the Lord to help us. Do you remember how the apostles asked the Lord to increase their faith? There are many stories of people of God who struggled at times to trust God. When we ask God to help us with our doubt, it gives him permission to work in our lives, increasing our faith.

(!) Consider the story of the boy possessed by a demonic spirit from his early childhood (see Mark 9:14 – 29). The father was weak in faith, but he asked Jesus to help his son. The father said, "But *if* you can do anything, have compassion on us and help us." And Jesus said to him, "*If you can*! All things are possible for one who believes." Immediately the father of the child cried out and said, "*I believe; help my unbelief!*"

This man cried out to Jesus in doubt, but Jesus responded to him that it would be possible if he would believe. The father realized his doubt. He told Jesus he believed and asked for help with his unbelief. Jesus made it a point to show this man that it is **not** about what **Jesus** could do. (After all, Jesus was given all authority in heaven and earth. See Matthew 28:18). It was about what the man could do. **Could he believe?** The man wanted the kind of faith that pleased Jesus and asked Him to help with his unbelief. Jesus honored his effort to trust, meeting him where he was, and He healed the boy. He will do the same for us. He meets us in our unbelief.

*Never hesitate to pray for help when you struggle with doubt and unbelief!*

## Denial

Denial is not the same as doubt. In denial, you refuse to look at part of yourself or your life honestly. This is a detrimental coping skill. Denial can show itself many ways:

- By minimizing a difficult time of life as being in the past and over, without ever addressing how it made us feel or the way it impacted how we respond to situations today.

- By ignoring a character flaw ("I'm not so bad; at least I'm not like_____!")

- By hiding a sin or issue in our family because of shame and embarrassment

- By drawing attention to another's flaws to draw attention away from our own issues

- By projecting negativity

- By burying how we feel in medication, illegal drugs, or alcohol

### Questions to Ponder

2.1) Make a plan to help grow your faith. Include studying the Word, how you will pray, and what you will do during a trial. Put your plan into action this week.

2.2) How are you going about daily praying and journaling? If you struggle to do this every day, write how you are struggling and a plan to help you be more consistent.

## Forget the Past

We should **not** hang onto the past, but the only way to truly overcome it is to deal with it. Then we can move ahead, leaving the pain of the past behind us. Paul says in Philippians 3:13,

> *Brothers, I do not consider that I have made it my own. But one thing I do:*
> *forgetting what lies behind and straining forward to what lies ahead.*

Some people use this verse as a reason not to dig up the past, thinking that doing so is merely being a victim, continually obsessed with what has happened to them. However, Paul is telling us to keep our eyes on where we are going, instead of looking back to where we have been. **He is not telling us to ignore the past**.

---

When you are in denial, refusing to look at or deal
with the things that hurt you in the past,
there are lasting consequences.

The result is that you cannot move forward, and
**you are in fact living in the oppression of your past,**
regardless of whether you can admit it or not.

Refusing to deal with past situations leaves you trapped there.

---

**Hanging onto our past is not always something we do knowingly!**

## Consequences of Denial

When you deny or discount your feelings, all your emotions become muted. Suppressed emotions can cause anxiety, expressing themselves as unexplainable fear and fatigue. Not only do we mute the bad feelings; we also silence the good ones. This can lead to depression. There is freedom in experiencing our emotions, even when the feelings are unpleasant.

Denial is as if you are running away from your past
yet terrified of stepping into your future.

### Questions to Ponder

2.3) **Can you identify coping skills that you use now (or have used in the past) to deal with shame, fear, pain, insecurity, depression, etc.? How do you handle difficult situations?**

2.4) **What have you clung to for way too long? Anger? Fear? Loneliness? Unforgiveness? Resentments? Or something else?**

Many people do not realize they have unmet expectations. Denial of your expectations may cause tension in your relationships and make you feel impatient and irritated. Even when you get what you thought you wanted, you still may not feel satisfied or find yourself complaining that nothing works out. Your denial causes you to live in the lie that you can somehow achieve the unreasonable expectations you place on yourself.

Denial is the lie that keeps us trapped **indefinitely**. It tells us we are safe from our past with our "yuck" buried behind vast walls no one can penetrate. But the people who have "walked in your shoes" can see right through those walls.

*In denial, we think we are hidden, but we are simply blind.*

Have you ever heard the saying, "You are only as sick as your secrets"? Your secrets are anything you deny and keep hidden in the dark. Bring those secrets into the light, and they lose their power over you. God promises us that while we are blind and stuck, He will guide us out of our darkness.

*And I will lead the blind in a way that they do not know, in paths that they have not known I will guide them. I will turn the darkness before them into light, the rough places into level ground. These are the things I do, and I do not forsake them.*
*(Isaiah 42:16)*

## Questions to Ponder

2.5) Fear can take many forms: Jealousy, insecurity, anxiety, worry, control, etc. In what ways do you experience fear?

2.6) Consider recent situations where you were wronged or felt uncomfortable. What was your emotional response? (Did you feel insecure, angry, fearful, panicked, sad/depressed, lonely/empty, numb, etc.?)

2.7) Take an honest look at yourself. Can you identify the walls you present to others?

2.8) What are your secrets? (These can include family secrets.) Bring them into the light!

---

**Today, commit to breaking out of your walls of denial.**

**Pray and speak to the Lord about your choice.**
**Ask him to search your heart and show you anything you missed.**

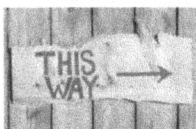

---

**Do you struggle to pray and journal?**
**Ask your coach to help you come up with a**
**plan to be consistent!**

# Chapter Three

## Surrender

# Lesson 3 — Why Surrender?

## Surrender

Most likely, if you are on this journey, you have been trying to get your life under control and finally decided to do something different. You will get a grip on your life once and for all!

What if, to gain a grip on your life, you had to loosen your grip on it?
Does that sound counter-productive—even crazy—to you?

**The two principal reasons we refuse to surrender are pride and control.** Pride separates us from God, and He expects us to give Him control.

Surrender is letting go, but what does that really mean? How does that work? Before you can let something go, you must identify what you are holding on to. Start examining how you handle life now. **Take your time** to answer these questions about your life and **answer as honestly** as you can.

We have discussed how faith is crucial for our relationship with God and our journey. Surrender is also crucial. **God is a gentleman.** He takes nothing you are not willing to give.

### Questions to Ponder

3.1) In what areas of your life are you holding onto regret? (Had I only made a different choice, everything would be different … )

3.2) What things have you been doing again and again in an effort to improve your life?

3.3) When have you made poor choices because your emotions led you, and what was the result?

3.4) What kinds of things have you done to ease or lessen pain in your heart?

3.5) List the things about which you are currently (or most) angry and resentful. How are these things affecting your life?

3.6) Where are you getting your purpose and value?

3.7) List all the positive labels that describe you. (Smart, beautiful, artist, designer, etc.)

3.8) List all the negative labels that describe you. (Stupid, fat, lazy, unpopular, rejected, selfish, ugly, etc.)

3.9) In what ways are you selfish or prone to putting yourself before others?

## Control

Control prevents surrender. Why do we refuse God access to part of our life, and fight Him for control? We covet control because we want things our way. We do not trust that God's way is best or that it will please us. We may fear His desires will not match our own, or that He may ask of us something we are not willing to give. Yet when we give over control, life becomes easier as we lose the burden of that responsibility. Complete surrender means we no longer need to worry because God will provide our needs. If we walk and abide with Him, we **will** do right by Him.

*I am the vine; you are the branches. Whoever abides in me and I in him, he it is that*
*bears much fruit, for apart from me you can do nothing. (John 15:5)*

## Powerless

In your flesh, you are powerless to do what is right and will always fall into sin. In your own wisdom, you will mess up every time. Your flesh pursues pleasure, often in sin, but happiness from worldly pursuits is always temporary. It lasts only a moment before you need to find something even bigger and greater to make you happy, and that too is short-lived. **The flesh can never be satisfied.** It will always want more and leave us searching our entire lives for fleeting moments of rest and happiness.

## Strength and Wisdom

The Lord gives us joy, which is better than happiness. Bad things happen to both "good" and "bad" people. With the Lord's joy in our lives, we can ride out life's storms in peace. Joy does not end, but happiness does. **You can have joy in difficult moments, even when you cannot have happiness.** The joy of the Lord gives us the strength, the ability to persevere and the desire to be and do more.

Wisdom is another source of strength in the Lord. In our own wisdom we only understand in part, from our limited perspective. We misunderstand people, become offended, fall into traps, and fail. However, the Lord knows everyone's heart. He sees the past, present, and future. He knows the beginning and the end of every situation you find yourself in, and the Lord always speaks truth. To live in His wisdom is to be strong in your life.

*Why would you ever want to use your own wisdom?*
*Why would you not want to give over control?*

---

## ! God Has Expectations

There are several things God expects from us. The most important are to **have faith** (trust), and **to surrender** to His will (give Him control). The more faith we have, the easier it is to give up our control. We must **relinquish our shortcomings** (sin and strongholds), so we can see clearly to help other believers do the same. It is through God that we overcome strongholds.

*You hypocrite, first take the log out of your own eye, and then*
*you will see clearly to take the speck out of your brother's eye. (Matthew 7:5)*

**He expects** our trust and obedience, that we will judge others fairly, and offer people forgiveness when they hurt us. These four things develop in us **a heart like Christ, full of love**, and love is the point of everything. Without love we are nothing. *(1 Corinthians 13:3).*

---

3.10) What do you have control over in your life?

3.11) In what areas do you lack control?

3.12) Are there areas of your life that you fear giving God control over? List them. For each item, describe what you are afraid of.

## Do we have control?

There is exceptionally little that we control. Most circumstances in life come about because of other people's choices, the government, or natural disasters (storms, fire, etc.), or any number of other causes. Out of everything we think we can control, we will find we can only control two things:

We have control over our thoughts and our choices. That is all!

In the previous questions, you may have mentioned situations where you are "in charge," such as if you manage employees at your work. The fact is that you may oversee your employees or children, but do you really have control over them? You can make choices to discipline them, to coerce compliance, but the choice to listen to your authority is theirs. You cannot control their choices. There really is not much we can control on this earth. We can possibly influence things and people, but we cannot control them.

Question to Ponder

3.13) What areas of your life are you willing to release your grip on and hand over to the Lord?

3.14) Review the "Stop, Drop, and Roll" strategy on the next page, and use it this week. Then write about how well it worked for you or about any difficulties using the strategy.

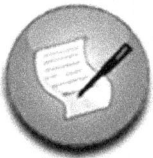

---

- **Do not forget to write about your day each evening in your journal.**
- **Write about areas of your life that have been holding you down.**
- **Write about unreasonable expectations or control issues you may have.**
- **Spend some quiet time studying the Word.**
- **Ask the Lord what He wants you to Surrender to Him.**

## Strategy: Stop, Drop, and Roll

Every bad choice begins with a wrong thought. It may seem difficult to believe that you have control over your thoughts, but you do—and stopping wrong thinking is vital to your recovery! You may not be able to stop a thought from entering your mind, but you can control how that thought affects you. The Word says to take your thoughts captive and make them obedient to the Lord. This implies that you should be aware of your thoughts. Dismiss wrong thinking and replace those thoughts with God's truth.

This strategy can help you prevent a crisis in any situation before it starts. Remember your fire safety lessons from school? They taught you if you are on fire, you must stop where you are, drop to the ground, and roll to smother the fire. Instead of a physical fire, we are going to teach you to put out symbolic fires in your thinking that can cause devastating burns.

## Stop

**Stop and think.** No matter what situation comes up, stop and think before you act. Stay aware of your thoughts throughout the day. Pay attention to emotional responses and see if you can identify the thought behind the response. What are you thinking? Is your self-talk detrimental? Are you leaning on the Lord in the situation, or on your own strength?

## Drop

**Drop the lie.** If you find your thinking goes against what you are learning from the Lord, you are on "fire." Identify the lie. Would the Lord say the same thing to you that you are saying to yourself? Would you give another person the advice you are speaking to yourself? Are your thoughts degrading you or another person? Test the thought with Scripture!

## Roll

**Roll with the truth.** Find the truth in the situation. Are you misunderstanding something? Pray for understanding and the Lord's wisdom on what to do. If you are distraught, seek the peace of the Lord through worship. Sometimes the lies in our mind shout so loudly they drown out the truth. If you must, shout the truth aloud until it is louder than the lies in your mind. You may get some strange looks, but it works!

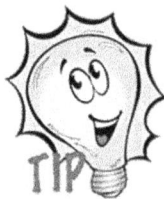

---

If you are unsure of God's truth for a particular situation, you can use tools such as

**https://www.openbible.info/**

to search Scripture for any topic you can imagine. Pray and ask the Holy Spirit to reveal the truth to you.

# Lesson 4 — Identifying Expectations

## Expectations

Expectations are some of the most **difficult things to surrender.** Everyone has expectations. We have expected things of people and carried the burden of other's expectations since we were young children. Sometimes we expect too much of ourselves, and other times we wear ourselves down trying to meet another person's unreasonable expectations. We may experience guilt when failing to live up to standards another sets, and sometimes we believe even God expects more than we can give. Examining expectations will help you discover areas you need to surrender.

Sometimes people want so much from us that it becomes a stress on our daily lives. We must learn to identify unfair expectations but **realize that not all expectations are harmful.** They may keep us motivated and accountable and help us set goals or make plans.

> ### Question to Ponder
> 4.1) Who places expectations on you? What are those expectations? (Be sure to include family, church, pastors, employers, friends, coworkers, and everyone you interact with regularly.)

## Expectations of self

When our expectations of ourselves are too high to meet, we may feel like a failure or that we cannot be good enough. Are you expecting perfection of yourself? Do you expect to accomplish more than your time allows? Are any of your expectations unnecessary? If you expect more of yourself than you can give, **especially** if others do **not** hold you to the same standard, you must evaluate your expectations.

Sometimes **we do not expect enough** from ourselves. This does not necessarily imply laziness, but it may indicate that you feel that you are not smart enough, talented enough, brave enough, or good enough to meet a higher expectation. Are there areas of your life where you should expect more of yourself?

Evaluate this carefully. Would you hold others to the same
expectations you set for yourself, or do you expect more
from others than you are willing to give?

Do you expect people to be your security, approval, value, purpose, confidence, love, or trust? Do others expect this of you? If you expect another to fill these holes in your life, you may blame them for your lack. In truth, you cannot count on another person to fill these gaps. People are flawed, and they are not designed to meet these needs. Eventually, they will fail you. If another expects this from you, you will fail them. These needs are holes in our life that can only be filled by God—the only one who will never fail.

## Analyze Your Expectations

Think about the expectations you identified in question 4.1. Try to see the reason behind these expectations from the other person's perspective. Is the expectation a responsibility to your family or a boss? Does the expectation have a positive impact or benefit on your life? **These are most likely reasonable expectations.**

On the other hand, do other people's expectations arise from selfish motives or take advantage of you? Are they more than you can give? Are the expectations placed on you different from the expectations placed on another in your position? Is it something another person would consider unfair or unreasonable if you asked them to do the same thing? If you said "yes" to any of these questions, **then they are probably unreasonable expectations.**

## Questions to Ponder

4.2) Think about the expectations you identified in question 4.1 from the other person's perspective. Are any of these expectations unreasonable?

4.3) Are these expectations hurting you (physically, emotionally, spiritually)? Describe How.

4.4) How should you handle these unreasonable expectations?

4.5) Now consider the expectations you put on yourself. Write a complete list of these expectations. Who else expects you to achieve these expectations?

4.6) What personal expectations should you reevaluate?

4.7) In what areas of your life can and should you expect more from yourself?

4.8) In what areas of your life do you lack confidence? How could you strengthen confidence in yourself?

4.9) Do you blame any of your problems on things that are missing from your life? What are those things?

4.10) What or who have you used to fill those gaps in your life?

# Lesson 5 — Down with Pride

There are many other reasons we refused to hand control over to God. Here are some that might sound familiar:

- We want things our own way. We want what we want, and we do not want God to do something different.
- We enjoy our sin and do not want to change it.
- We worry about what others will think about us or what we are doing.
- We are afraid. A common first response to fear is to want to take control.
- We assume we know what is best.

These ways of thinking are birthed by fear and pride. Fear is a lie of the enemy. We fear not having what we want or losing opportunities. Sometimes we fear we will miss out on something fun. We fear people's opinions because we are afraid to offend and fear rejection. We think we know better, and that listening to God or another's advice will not produce our desired result. We need not be afraid. God can take better care of us and our loved ones than we ever could.

## Pride

**Pride is not just thinking more of yourself than you should. It manifests in many ways.** Most of us understand pride as when we think we have better, do better, or are better than another person. Pride is also when we think we are better, know better, or can do better than God. We display our pride many ways:

- Not following rules or laws
- Refusing to listen or hear sound counsel
- Being judgmental and comparing ourselves to others
- Seeking to control a situation
- Bossiness, or demanding that others think and act our way
- Conceit, arrogance, and self-praise
- Selfishness
- Vengefulness
- Teasing and mockery
- Gossip and seeking "dirt" on someone, or harboring evil suspicions
- Rejecting those in different economic, racial, political, or other groups
- Causing disputes about words to prove we are correct
- Stirring up controversial arguments, etc.

Have you ever met someone who often degrades themselves, cannot be comforted, speaks and acts like a victim, or constantly complains about how they are treated? These people, living in a state of continuous humiliation, may in fact be prideful, desiring praise and attention. Their false humility can be a form of manipulation to get others to feed their pride.

Pride prevents surrender and separates us from God. There are hundreds of scriptures dealing with pride or prideful behavior. Pride prevents us from having a proper relationship with the Lord. When we believe our wisdom is better than God's, we may become a stumbling block to others. Pride destroys people with words; it causes envy, strife, divisiveness, manipulation, and evil suspicions. God detests pride and resists the proud.

*You adulterous people! Do you not know that friendship with the world is enmity with God? Therefore whoever wishes to be a friend of the world makes himself an enemy of God... Therefore it says, "God opposes the proud but gives grace to the humble." Submit yourselves therefore to God. Resist the devil, and he will flee from you. Draw near to God, and he will draw near to you. (James 4:4 – 6)*

*Do nothing from selfish ambition or conceit, but in humility count others more significant than yourselves. Let each of you look not only to his own interests, but also to the interests of others. (Philippians 2:3 – 4)*

*When pride comes, then comes disgrace, but with the humble is wisdom. (Proverbs 11:2)*

*Do you see a man who is wise in his own eyes?
There is more hope for a fool than for him. (Proverbs. 26:12)*

## Questions to Ponder

5.1) Consider all the expressions of pride mentioned in this lesson. In what ways are you prideful?

5.2) Pray about surrender and pride. Is there something God is asking you to surrender?

5.3) Why does He want you to surrender this?

5.4) When we surrender something, we replace it with something else. With what are you replacing the things you have surrendered? How do you fill the empty places in your life?

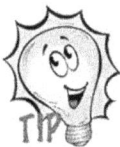

When we surrender something to the Lord, give up a harmful sin, or change a way of thinking, we may experience loss that leaves an empty place in our heart. God does not want that for us. He wants us to have joy! Surrender requires refilling!

Any gaps in your heart will be filled with something, so allow the Lord to fill those places. Seek His presence, read His Word, worship, and pray. A solid relationship with the Lord will begin to remove the loss or grief experienced from changes in our life.

# Lesson 6 — Giving Up

## It All Works Together

Throughout your journey, you will continue to find areas of denial, pride, and control that need to be surrendered to the Lord. Now that you understand how to identify them, it will be easier to give issues to God as they come up. Each evening, as you journal about your day, think about how control and pride are evident in your life.

## What Is Surrender, and How Do I Do it?

Surrender is giving up control, laying down your pride, and being obedient to the Lord. It is vital for your journey. It sacrifices your selfish desires and changes your heart to accept God's will as your own. Surrender is coming to the end of self-effort and giving up. **It is giving up your time, will, emotions, and life to the Lord.** God wants us to live in **a state of constant surrender** to Him, a constant state of giving up to Him so He can direct our every step.

*I know, O LORD, that the way of man is not in himself,*
*that it is not in man who walks to direct his steps. (Jeremiah 10:23)*

We are to deny our own desires and will for His.

*And he said to all, "If anyone would come after me, let him deny himself and take up*
*his cross daily and follow me. For whoever would save his life will lose it, but*
*whoever loses his life for my sake will save it." (Luke 9:23 – 24)*

## How Do We Surrender?

We are promised increase when we first seek God's Kingdom, His ways, and right standing with Him. We must also abide in Him. This means we live in Him and His Spirit lives in us. Without Him, we can do nothing, but in Him we can do all things. If your first priority is to seek His kingdom, you will have all that you need.

*But seek first the kingdom of God and his righteousness, and all these things*
*will be added to you. (Matthew 6:33)*

*Abide in me, and I in you. As the branch cannot bear fruit by itself, unless it abides in the*
*vine, neither can you, unless you abide in me. I am the vine; you are the branches. Whoever*
*abides in me and I in him, he it is that bears much fruit, for apart from me you can do*
*nothing. If anyone does not abide in me he is thrown away like a branch and withers; and*
*the branches are gathered, thrown into the fire, and burned. If you abide in me, and my*
*words abide in you, ask whatever you wish, and it will be done for you. (John 15:4 – 7)*

**Surrender is:**

- To allow the Lord access into an area of your life
- To give up your own control and desire in that area
- To give the Lord permission to do with it what He wants
- To allow the Lord to control the outcome

When you surrender something to the Lord, the burden of the result rests on Him, not you!

## Surrender Displayed through the Life of Moses

In the book of Exodus, God approached Moses, manifested as a burning bush.

> *"Come, I will send you to Pharaoh that you may bring my people, the children of Israel, out of Egypt." But Moses said to God, "Who am I that I should go to Pharaoh and bring the children of Israel out of Egypt?" ... Then Moses said to God, "If I come to the people of Israel and say to them, 'The God of your fathers has sent me to you'" and they ask me, 'What is his name?' what shall I say to them?" God said to Moses, "I AM WHO I AM." And he said, "Say this to the people of Israel: 'I AM has sent me to you."*
> *(Exodus 3:10 – 11, 13 – 14)*

Moses asked who he was to serve, and then who God was. God answered, "I AM WHO I AM." It was never about Moses or his ability to serve; **it was about God**. We do not need to be in control, because God is. **In fact, there cannot be two "I AMs" in control.** You cannot say, "I am in control of my life" and also say, "The I AM is in control of my life." One must yield. Will you keep a tight hold on your control, or give control over to the Lord?

## How Do I Know What Needs to Be Surrendered? What if I Am in Denial?

One way to identify what you need to give up is to look at the causes of your anger. At times, anger is justified; many times, however, anger is an indicator of a larger issue. For instance, conversation topics that are "off-limits" because you fear how you may respond may indicate denial or something you have not fully surrendered. Sometimes we cannot understand why we do what we do. It is easier to see from an outside perspective. You may need to ask your coach, accountability partner, or **someone you respect** for his or her perspective and be **willing to hear it with an open mind**.

> ### Questions to Ponder
> 6.1) In what ways have you tried to control the outcome of situations?
>
> 6.2) What did you compromise or lose to achieve that outcome?
>
> 6.3) What things do people say or do to make you feel defensive? What life circumstances put you on the defensive?
>
> 6.4) What are the things people say or do that make you angry? What life circumstances make you angry?
>
> 6.5) What topics are not open for discussion with you? Can you spot areas in your life where being angry or threatened show something you should surrender?

# Lesson 7 — Trust

## Surrender Requires Trust

When we place more faith and trust in ourselves than in our God, we do not feel safe to surrender. **Trust is the crucial element that makes surrender possible** and allows a heart change. At first, trusting is difficult, but the Lord knows this and makes a way. Give Him your mustard seed of trust and watch God make it grow. Some tough situations can leave us wondering where God is. Our faith shows us that He is, in fact, there. God's Word says that He will never leave us. Just because you cannot see how He is working doesn't mean that He isn't.

> *Cast your burden on the Lord, and he will sustain you;*
> *he will never permit the righteous to be moved. (Psalm 55:22)*

When we become distracted, we move away from the Lord. Fear and anger make it difficult to see His work. Even when we cannot experience His presence, however, He is there. He grieves over the things that break our hearts. He sees our struggles, pain, wrong thinking, and discouragement, and He is always working in the background. The enemy makes plans to destroy us, but every time God turns them for our good. You can count on this truth.

> *As for you, you meant evil against me, but God meant it for good, to bring it about that many*
> *people should be kept alive, as they are today. (Genesis 50:20)*

## The Result of Faith and Surrender Is a Transformed Heart and Changed Life

**Surrender allows God to work.** He is the one who changes our hearts, gives us increase, and takes us from one measure of glory to the next. This lifelong process promises the result that we will be complete and whole.

> *And we all, with unveiled face, beholding the glory*
> *of the Lord, are being transformed into the same*
> *image from one degree of glory to another. For*
> *this comes from the Lord who is the Spirit.*
> *(2 Corinthians 3:18)*

> *And let steadfastness have its full effect, that you*
> *may be perfect and complete, lacking in nothing.*
> *(James 1:4)*

> *And I am sure of this, that he who began a good*
> *work in you will bring it to completion at the day*
> *of Jesus Christ. (Philippians 1:6)*

> *And have put on the new self, which is being*
> *renewed in knowledge after the image of its*
> *creator. (Colossians 3:10)*

---

Can you extend trust to God just for today?

**Allow Him to prove Himself faithful to you.**

## He will!

**Then tomorrow, do it again!**

You will begin growing in an unshakable faith in the Lord!

**Here is how God changes our hearts:**

- We believe God will save us and change our lives.

- We offer God our trust in a difficult situation.

- God proves himself trustworthy.

- We trust God over and over, and He proves His faithfulness, increasing our faith and trust in Him.

- We love God because He loves us.

- Our love transforms our desires to become more like what He desires.

- We cry out, asking Him to change what we cannot change.

- We allow God in, and then He changes our hearts and our lives. (He will not come in without our permission. We have a free will to choose His ways!)

## How Do You Overcome Fear to Trust?

Imagine a mother whose teenage daughter is an addict. Even when the girl is clean, Mom cannot trust she will not lie or steal from her. This is what she has always done. She gets clean for a while, a month, maybe a year, and then it begins again. The lying starts. Mom does not know where her daughter is or what she is doing, and she is terrified she will find her daughter dead one day. Then Mom's good jewelry goes missing, along with money from her purse. The girl gets help and tries life again, but eventually fails, and the cycle begins again. It has been the same story for years.

This time, however, is different. The daughter is making an honest effort and trying hard to earn trust again, but how can her mom ever trust her? Yet if her mom never gives her trust, then she can never overcome. Her failure will always condemn her. She will never rise above her "addict" label, but Mom is afraid to trust. She cannot cope with the pain and fear of losing her daughter.

> 1 Corinthians 13 equates love with trusting (believing). Trust is a sacrifice.
> It is a genuine act of love to allow yourself to become vulnerable.

This time, Mom does something different, too. She chooses to tell her daughter that today she will extend trust to her and see what happens. The daughter proves herself trustworthy, and Mom is pleased. Each day, she extends that gift of trust to her daughter, and each day she grows more confident in her. Eventually, she will no longer worry about her daughter failing. By trusting her daughter, Mom gives her the encouragement she needs to continue trying and doing right.

**The secret is offering trust even when you believe the person, or even God, may fail you,** and giving them the opportunity to prove they are trustworthy. **Trust is a gift of redemption.**

*Note: There are times when it is not recommended to extend trust. You do not know if someone is ready to change their life, but God does! Listen for His wisdom. Ask your coach for additional resources.*

*Without the opportunity to fail, there is no opportunity to succeed.*

## Questions to Ponder

7.1) What places in your life do you now trust to hand over to God?

7.2) Is there a time in your life where God failed you? What happened? Whose choices were responsible for what happened?

7.3) Write *every time* you can remember in which God has been there for you, encouraged you or given you strength to get through an impossible situation.

7.4) Are you angry with God? Why?

7.5) Are you willing to give God a chance to prove Himself trustworthy to you?

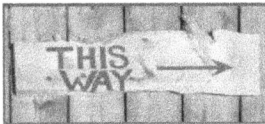

**Work with your coach to seek answers regarding your anger or disappointment with God.**

# Chapter Four

# God's Expectations
# & Commitment

# *Lesson 8 — Broken Expectations*

8.1) We all have expectations of God. What do you expect of Him?

## When God Disappoints Our Expectations

God tells us what we can expect from Him when we follow His ways. He will never let us down and never leave us. He meets us where we are. All He asks in return is our trust (faith) and a heart surrendered, seeking truth, willing to examine flaws, and open to being changed. God always has our best interests in mind, even if it does not always feel that way.

Misconceptions about God cause wrong expectations that lead to disappointment. When we lean too much on one characteristic of God or one part of Scripture, misunderstandings will happen. For example, if you lean too much on God's grace and ignore repentance, you may feel abandoned when you suffer the natural consequence of your sin. Likewise, if you lean too much on your works and service, you may miss relationship with God. The truth becomes skewed when we do not see the entire picture. Clarification comes when we consider the whole counsel of God's word.

If you draw two perfectly parallel lines on a piece of paper, you could continue the lines out forever, and they will never get farther apart. What if, instead, when you started to draw those lines, you were off by 0.01°? To the naked eye, the lines would appear to be parallel. As the lines are drawn out, however, they would get farther and farther away from each other. Apply this same concept to the Word of God. A small misunderstanding at the beginning can drive you further away until the truth is unrecognizable. This is why it is vital to understand how all of Scripture works together to show one complete truth.

## Our Expectations of God

How do you know if your expectations of God are wrong? How do you respond when your prayers are not answered the way you expect? What happens when your faith is shaken? These questions can help identify what you are expecting from God. When God's answers seem unfair, we can find our faith shaken. Then one of three things happens:

1) **We doubt God's word.** Some people completely reject God because they feel He "didn't come through" or "allowed them to be hurt."

2) **We assume we have done something wrong that prevents God from helping us.** We sin too much or believe too little. Either way, this thinking leads to the same place: a belief that "I am not enough."

3) **We know God is good and wants what is best for us, so there must be something we missed or cannot yet see.** This is a good place to be. This understanding allows us to seek the Lord for answers and be patient for His response.

## God Has Expectations of Us

God's plan to heal is taking away our sins and giving us new life in Him. It begins with our confession of faith, the blood of Jesus removing our sin. Then the process of **transformation into new life begins as we develop a relationship with God**. This process involves more than knowing the Scripture. It includes applying the Word of God in our lives. It is allowing the Lord into the dark places of our hearts to root out the damage, so we can put on a new identity in Him. This process requires surrender, since the Lord will not take what we will not freely give. Relationship is reciprocal, meaning that each person gives and receives from the other. Our healing is a cooperative effort with God. He has expectations of His people.

**What are God's expectations?** God expects that we:

- Trust and surrender control, giving the Lord permission to work in our heart
- Look at current and past situations with God's perspective
- Learn God's Word, pray, seek a relationship with Him, love Him, and listen to Him
- Pull the walls down from around our heart
- Examine our heart and remove character flaws that displease the Lord
- Put off our old self, old ways, old desires, and our past
- Guard our thoughts and make them obedient to Christ and His truth
- Share the hope we find in Jesus with others

*Now this I say and testify in the Lord, that you must no longer walk as the Gentiles do, in the futility of their minds. They are darkened in their understanding, alienated from the life of God because of the ignorance that is in them, due to their hardness of heart. They have become callous and have given themselves up to sensuality, greedy to practice every kind of impurity. But that is not the way you learned Christ!—assuming that you have heard about him and were taught in him, as the truth is in Jesus, to put off your old self, which belongs to your former manner of life and is corrupt through deceitful desires, and to be renewed in the spirit of your minds, and to put on the new self, created after the likeness of God in true righteousness and holiness.*
*(Ephesians 4:17 – 24)*

### Questions to Ponder

8.2) In the past or present, what beliefs seem to have failed you?

8.3) Are your answers to question 8.2 based in truth? Search the Scripture to discover the truth according to God's word.

8.4) Are all your expectations of God reasonable? Why or why not?

8.5) Reread the list of expectations God has of us. Which expectations do you meet?

8.6) Do you object to, neglect, or misunderstand any of God's expectations?

# Lesson 9 — Expect Transformation

## You Can Expect a Transformed, New Life!

*Count it all joy, my brothers, when you meet trials of various kinds, for you know that the testing of your faith produces steadfastness. And let steadfastness have its full effect, that you may be perfect and complete, lacking in nothing. (James 1:2 – 4)*

You can expect a journey with God to transform your life into a better life in Christ. You probably believe Antarctica exists even though you have never been there to see it, yet that belief doesn't change your life. But the result of a belief in Jesus is a transformed life. The proof of transformation is the fruit demonstrated in a person's life (see Matthew 7:16). This fruit is not simply moral behavior but transformed character: love, joy, self-control, patience, kindness, goodness, gentleness, faithfulness, and peace. God's spirit is evident in a transformed heart, but transformation is a process.

*We know that our old self was crucified with him in order that the body of sin might be brought to nothing, so that we would no longer be enslaved to sin. For one who has died has been set free from sin. Now if we have died with Christ, we believe that we will also live with him. (Romans 6:6 – 8)*

## You Can Expect Help

You can call on the Lord to help you with anything you face. He is your healer, counselor, and protector. He helps you grow spiritually. He increases your faith, teaches you His truth, and convicts you of wrong.

*So we can confidently say, "The Lord is my helper; I will not fear; what can man do to me?" (Hebrews 13:6)*

*But the Helper, the Holy Spirit, whom the Father will send in my name, he will teach you all things and bring to your remembrance all that I have said to you. (John 14:26)*

## You Can Expect God to Be Patient with You

The Lord knows your beginning, your end, and all the choices you make in between. He knows the path you choose for your life, your ups and downs, and your right and wrong choices. He has great patience with you, disciplining and guiding you in gentle love to ensure your future with Him. He meets you where you are and leads you from there. You do not need to be good enough to seek God, and in fact your effort cannot make you righteous. Your sin nature corrupts your goodness so you cannot be good enough for God, but you are so valuable to God that he created a way to make you "good enough" through Christ's sacrifice.

*The Lord is not slow to fulfill his promise as some count slowness, but is patient toward you, not wishing that any should perish, but that all should reach repentance. (2 Peter 3:9)*

## You Can Expect Hope, Purpose, and a Future

God has declared that His plans for you will be to your benefit. He gives you purpose, both here and in eternity. He raises you from "glory to glory" to prepare you for His plans. Your purpose on earth gives you hope and prepares you for your eternal purpose. You can trust God to help you find and fulfill that purpose.

*For I know the plans I have for you, declares the Lord, plans for welfare and not for evil, to give you a future and a hope. (Jeremiah 29:11)*

## You Can Expect Love

As you surrender your control and fear, you become open to knowing and loving God. In return, you receive a love and acceptance from God that penetrates your heart. His love gives you confidence, approval, a sense of wellbeing, and freedom from the opinions of others.

*So, we have come to know and to believe the love that God has for us. God is love, and whoever abides in love abides in God, and God abides in him. (1 John 4:16)*

## You Can Expect Freedom

What does freedom look like? It is abundant life in the Lord. It is casting your fear, anxiety, and worry on the Lord, lightening the load you must carry. Freedom is knowing who God is and who you are in Him. It is wielding truth to escape the guilt and shame of sin, past mistakes, and wrong choices. It is tearing down walls, discovering a new identity, and removing chains of pain and loss that keep you trapped in your own personal prison.

*The Spirit of the Lord God is upon me, because the Lord has anointed me to bring good news to the poor; he has sent me to bind up the brokenhearted, to proclaim liberty to the captives, and the opening of the prison to those who are bound. (Isaiah 61:1)*

*So Jesus said to the Jews who had believed him, "If you abide in my word, you are truly my disciples, and you will know the truth, and the truth will set you free. … Truly, truly, I say to you, everyone who practices sin is a slave to sin. The slave does not remain in the house forever; the son remains forever. So if the Son sets you free, you will be free indeed." (John 8:31 – 32, 34 – 36)*

## You Can Expect God to Protect and Fight

As you begin your journey, the enemy may attack you with doubt, fear, angry thoughts, family issues, financial struggles, or anything else he can throw in your way. He will fight to keep his grip on you, but you are headed toward freedom. The Lord fights for you. A spiritual battle is taking place on your behalf. **Do not hesitate to call on God every time a situation seems too much for you to handle.** God turns every trial to your benefit. No struggle is wasted. He turns the enemy's plans against him. Be still and let God work.

*No weapon that is fashioned against you shall succeed, and you shall confute every tongue that rises against you in judgment. This is the heritage of the servants of the Lord and their vindication from me, declares the Lord. (Isaiah 54:17)*

*The Lord will fight for you, and you have only to be silent. (Exodus 14:14)*

## You Can Expect Strength

When you are weak, unable to handle life, you find strength in the Lord. You find rest when you call on Him. Your weakness makes God shine. This is where He does His greatest work!

*Fear not, for I am with you; be not dismayed, for I am your God; I will strengthen you,*
*I will help you, I will uphold you with my righteous right hand. (Isaiah 41:10)*

*But he said to me, "My grace is sufficient for you, for my power is made perfect in*
*weakness." Therefore I will boast all the more gladly of my weaknesses, so that*
*the power of Christ may rest upon me. (2 Corinthians 12:9)*

## You Can Expect the Lord to Keep You

The Lord will not let you fall during your journey with Him. He will hold on to you and keep you on the right path when you falter. He will walk with you to the degree you allow Him, and sometimes He will even carry you. Hold Him tight, and He will keep a tight hold on you!

*The Lord will keep your going out and your coming in from this time forth and forevermore.*
*(Psalm 121:8)*

*Keep me as the apple of your eye; hide me in the shadow of your wings. (Psalm 17:8)*

## We Can Expect Relationship

When God reveals Himself to us He uses relational titles to show His desire for relationship with us. You are His beloved, His bride, His child, His friend, His servant. Relationship requires communication. Your heart speaks to Him in your prayers, and He communicates through His Spirit and written word, giving understanding and wisdom. Sometimes, He speaks through spiritual gifts. He teaches His people to hear His voice. You can expect to hear God speak.

*Draw near to God, and he will draw near to you. (James 4:8a)*

## You Can Expect to Overcome

Nowhere does Scripture promise a trouble-free life. It says **all** will have trouble, believers and non-believers alike. The believer, however, has assurance that God is with him, and there is nothing God cannot handle. Jesus overcame the world, and in Him, you will too.

*I have said these things to you, that in me you may have peace. In the world you will have*
*tribulation. But take heart; I have overcome the world. (John 16:33)*

## You Can Expect Joy

Remember, there is a difference between joy and happiness. God brings you to a place where you can live in His joy. Joy is the ability not to worry or fear. When you give God your problems, pain, and fears, His joy penetrates your heart.

*So also you have sorrow now, but I will see you again, and your hearts will rejoice,*
*and no one will take your joy from you. (John 16:22)*

## You Can Expect Perfect Peace

Peace directly results from trust, and trust comes as you keep your mind on God's protection and provision. Knowing God takes care of you, regardless of how it seems, brings perfect peace.

*You keep him in perfect peace whose mind is stayed on you, because he trusts in you.*
*(Isaiah 26:3)*

## We Can Expect a Heavenly Transplant

The power of God changes our heart. When our hardened heart breaks for Him, the Lord removes our stony heart and gives us a soft, pliable heart of flesh. He transforms us into His image like a caterpillar in a cocoon transforms into a new creation. Eventually, the caterpillar's struggle to break out of its walls ends, and a beautiful new life emerges. Your struggle too will end as the Lord breaks through your walls.

*And I will give them <u>one</u> heart, and a new spirit I will put within them. I will remove the heart of stone from their flesh and give them a heart of flesh. (Ezekiel 11:19)*

*Do not love the world or the things in the world. If anyone loves the world, the love of the Father is not in him. (1 John 2:15)*

### Questions to Ponder

9.1) According to the Scripture passages above, what results can you expect on this journey?

9.2) Which expectations mentioned in this chapter have you experienced with God?

9.3) Has God ever disappointed you by failing to meet a "reasonable" expectation?

9.4) Why has God not always answered your expectations as you wanted?

9.5) Our free will and the free will of others can become an obstacle to our recovery. Are you willing to surrender your will for the will of God with patience for His work to come to completion?

---

Your faith in His word (Jesus) activates the desire in God to act in your life, and your surrender activates God's power to act. As you overcome and see His awesome works, your desires change. You will likely long to learn more about Him and His ways. The more you see Him, the more you fall in love with Him. The more you love Him, the more obedient you become. The more you seek, the more He draws near. The more He draws near, the more you look like Him!

---

**Do not forget to write in your journal and Spend some quiet time with the Lord.**

*(Continue to Commitment)*

# Commitment

**It is important to stay committed to your journey.** If you give up, you will remain stuck and may even spiral into a deeper mess. It is also vital that you make a commitment to the Lord. This journey can only be taken hand-in-hand with Him. Only God can remove the damage caused by your sins and mistakes. Only He can heal your pain and set you free to be the person He created you to be.

**If you have never asked God to become your Lord and save you from your sins, would you like to do that now?** Do you believe in Jesus and trust Him (faith)? Are you willing to let Him be Lord in your life (willing to surrender to His will)?

## What is my commitment when I invite Jesus into my life?

You are committing to relationship with the Lord. He requires your faith. He expects you to turn to Him, listening for the Holy Spirit to teach you, so you can know God (and yourself) better. He expects you to live for Him, not for the approval of man, and to learn His voice.

He wants you to surrender to His ways, (obey) and seek after Him with all your heart. He rewards those who do this with promise after promise in Scripture. Ask Him to search your heart and show you any wicked way in you. He expects your prayers and gratitude for current and future blessings.

**Most importantly, He wants you to love Him!**

---

**(!) If you are ready … all you need to do is tell Him!**

Pray from your heart. **_To receive it, you must believe it!_** There is no specific "Sinner's Prayer" to receive salvation, but there are some things that you should include as you pray:

- Ask forgiveness for your sins.
- Claim your belief that Jesus is the Messiah who died to carry the burden of all your sins, and then He rose again.
- Trust Him to lead your life in the way you should go.
- Ask Him to become Lord of your life and invite His Spirit to live in your heart.

---

*"And without faith it is impossible to please him, for whoever would draw near to God must believe that he exists and that he rewards those who seek him." (Hebrews 11:6)*

*"Blessed is the man who remains steadfast under trial, for when he has stood the test he will receive the crown of life, which God has promised to those who love him." (James 1:12)*

*"You will seek me and find me, when you seek me with all your heart." (Jeremiah 29:13)*

*"Search me, O God, and know my heart! Try me and know my thoughts! And see if there be any grievous way in me, and lead me in the way everlasting!" (Psalm 139:23 – 24)*

*"For am I now seeking the approval of man, or of God? Or am I trying to please man? If I were still trying to please man, I would not be a servant of Christ." (Galatians 1:10)*

Visit the website at:

*www.rebuiltrecovery.org*

for downloadable pages and
more helpful resources!

www.ingramcontent.com/pod-product-compliance
Lightning Source LLC
Chambersburg PA
CBHW080425030426

42335CB00020B/2599